Bulletproof Diet

Delicious Recipes For The Bulletproof Diet To Remain Healthy And Feel Great

(Quick And Simple Weight Loss Recipes For The Bulletproof Diet)

Jean-Luc Desmarais

TABLE OF CONTENT

chapter 1: Awaken To A New Lifestyle 1

Bulletproof Coffee 3

Chapter 2: Why Grass-Fed Ingredients For The Bulletproof Diet? 5

Chapter 3: Rapid Protein Digestion 6

Chapter 4: How Does Weight Loss Typically Function? 13

Chapter 5: The Impact Of Physical Activity On Body Inflammation 18

Chapter 6: Imagine New Dreams 22

Chapter 7: How To Lose Weight On The Bulletproof Diet And Crucial Supplement Information 31

Smoothie With Cold Brew Colada And Bulletproof Coffee 44

Smoked Salmon And Avocado Are Delectable. 46

Season With A Pinch Of Sea Salt And Serve Immediately.Creamy Vegetables 47

Grass-Fed Lamb Prepared Moroccan-Style With Sweet And Sour Sprouts.................................. 49

Smoothie With Avocado And Raspberry........... 51

Baked Avocado N' Egg.. 55

Guacamole Impenetrable... 56

Coffee Made With Coconut Butter........................ 60

Buttery Broccoli... 64

Vanilla Cream Bulletproof....................................... 66

'Whatever' Exclaimed Tor Dnner......................... 68

Cauliflower Curry.. 70

Sausage-Burger Balls... 72

Eggs Scrambled With Spinach 74

Watercress Shake.. 77

Bulletproof Banana Pancakes 78

Chapter 1: Awaken To A New Lifestyle

The dawn reveals the day! Well, for me, the breakfast determines and shapes the day! You can attribute your diminishing energy levels throughout the day to the breakfast you chose in the morning. The primary culprits are the majority of the convenient food options that you are tempted to use so frequently. Modernity is characterized by stocking the pantry with ready-to-eat donuts and instant black coffee to rouse slumberous. Initially, these things may simple make you just feel satisfied and energized, but as the day progresses, they tend to simple make you just feel worse.

The sugar-laden cereals that you have been giving your children with such glee should be avoided at all costs. In addition, the frozen sausages and salamis that you deftly remove from your freezer to demonstrate your intelligence as a mother or hostess are also to blame. Because, in addition to ensuring that they taste great, are you aware of the quality of the meat used?

Knowing how much you enjoy your morning brew, here is the renowned Bulletproof Coffee that will provide you with much-needed energy and vitality. It contains grass-fed butter. And if that makes you twitch and squirm, believe me, I did the same thing when I first heard it. In harsh climates and high-altitude regions, however, this is the beverage of choice for sustaining high energy levels throughout the day. If you're concerned about the fats in butter, you should know that your body craves healthy fats, which this butter provides.

Bulletproof Coffee

- 1-5 Tablespoons Brain Octane Oil
- 1-5 Tablespoons grass-fed, unsalted butter or ghee
- 2 Cup filtered water
- 5 heaped teaspoons freshly ground Bulletproof Coffee Beans

1. Boil water for 1-5 minutes and add freshly ground coffee beans before turning the stove off.//
2. Then mix all other ingredients and simply put them in the blender for 50-90 seconds.
3. Pour the creamy, luscious coffee blend and enjoy.
4. All we did was to replace sugar with healthy fats and butter that would simple make your body replenished

with essential nutrients needed for the day.

5. Also it is going to simple make you just feel full for a longer duration without having to reach out for those unhealthy fatty snacks.

Chapter 2: Why Grass-Fed Ingredients For The Bulletproof Diet?

You've probably always heard that to lose weight, you must completely avoid butter and fats. However, this is because you are unaware of the benefits of grass-fed butter. This is derived from grass-fed rather than grain-fed cows. This enables them to produce fat that is significantly healthier than that obtained from cows fed corn and soy. This butter optimises the cholesterol level in the body and reduces it dramatically over time, making you "immune" to heart diseases for which cholesterol is the primary cause.

Chapter 3: Rapid Protein Digestion

Proten fasting entails abstaining from rroten for one week, consuming no more than 1,525 to 30 gramme. The reason we do this is because when a body doesn't have a script, it engages in auto-digestion, or elf- digestion. Indeed, that is exactly how it sounds. It means that your body uses the enzymes intended to digest protein to digest waste within your cells. Our sales assume waste and toxic waste, which slows us down and ages us. When we bohask our wau into autorhagu, we fight back, clearing away the body's waste and giving our sell a fresh start. Suddenly, uour body feels lighter, and your brain feels brighter.

If you really want to make it easier, choose the same day each week and just get into the habit of cooking on that day. Once you just get the hang of it,

Bulletproof Proten Fatng becomes just another part of your routine, and one that provides significant benefits when you're bulking. Here's how: Protein enhances cellular regenerative function. In addition to removing toxins, the enzymes from your pancreas and liver also remove debris from your spleen. Because autorhagu is the only known mechanism for regenerating mitochondria, proteins improve mitochondrial function. And when your sales performance improves, so will yours.

Proten fasting also improves your brain's ability to drain waste through the glumrhats utem and promotes better leer, which is an additional way to enhance your mental and rhual reerformanse.

You're probably wondering how you'll just get energy and feel full if you eliminate carbohydrates, but remember that you can just get an abundance of energy and satiety from good fats. Start the day with Bulletroof Coffee for a healthy dose of fats and caffeine, and then consume a diet rich in fats and moderate in carbohydrates throughout the day. You will find multiple protein-rich meal recipes in the index. For optimal results, limit carbohydrate consumption until later in the day, which improves the quality of the beer. It may sound simple, and it will be once you become accustomed to it, but be aware: Proteins lurk in unexplored regions. Broccoli? There is a rroten. You will also need to exercise caution when reserving space. According to the FDA, anything with less than 12 grammes of protein must be labelled as 0 grammes; therefore, you should monitor the amount of any food that may contain protein, even in trace amounts (vegetables and even soy milk, for example), as these foods may contain protein in amounts that are not listed on the label.

When it comes to bulletproofing yourself, resistance training is one of your most potent weapons. It's also great because you can use it on a routine basis, such as once per week, or when you're sick or have a compromised immune system. Utilize this tool to boost your singular function when you need it most. Autorhagu is also required to maintain muscle mass, as it inhibits catabolism. It prevents muscle deterioration in adults, so it makes your system perform better and your body look better.

As with any form of dieting or fasting, going overboard will likely have negative effects on your body and mind. If you become deficient in shronsallu rroten, your body will suffer. Insufficiency in protein will result in diminished immune function, muscle mass, and bone density, as well as diminished endurance. When I first began experimenting with protein fasting, I attempted to reduce my intake to 2,510 grammes per fasting day. But as I pushed myself further, I discovered that limiting my intake to 12 510 grammes per day produced the desired results—as long as I did so in limited quantities. I quickly cured my abdominal inflammation and ate a muffin. (Yes, even Bulletrroofer is susceptible to the dreaded muffin top once in a while!) Protein consumption feels like a deer bath that revitalises my entire body, right down to the cellular level. The secret is to bohask autorhagu in 248-hour bursts at a time. Thus, you receive all of the benefits without the negative side effects.

Bulletproof Proten fasting is not as simple as black and white. Everyone will respond to it differently and to varying degrees of intensity. Try varying amounts of writing to determine what works best for you. The essence of biohacking is discovering what works best for your body. The statement should exclude pregnant women, for whom neither intermittent nor protein fasting is a good idea. If you are eating for two, you must receive your food steadily. After a healthy birth, you can always ask the baby's weight.

Protective Proten Fasting is a biohack that reduces inflammation and kickstarts weight loss. For new readers and regular Bulletrroof followers. It is a day of protein fasting once per week in which you consume virtually no protein;

limit your daily protein intake to 12,510 grammes or less. To stay satiated and energised, consume a serving of Bulletrroof. Coffee in the morning and a diet of high fat, low protein, and moderate carbohydrates throughout the day. Limit sarbohudrate to afternoon and evening for optimal results.just get just get just keep

Chapter 4: How Does Weight Loss Typically Function?

What if I told you that losing weight is actually quite simple? You may believe that I have lost my mind. If you are like the majority of individuals who have struggled with their weight, "simple" is not the first word that comes to mind when describing dieting.

It is simple to become frustrated with weight loss. Many people struggle to lose weight and maintain their weight loss. In contrast, the human metabolism is relatively straightforward when viewed in the context of a large image of a human being.

In actuality, it can be reduced to a simple mathematical formula: calories consumed minus calories expended. When attempting to lose weight, you have only two options. It may appear that there are numerous options and systems for weight loss, but in reality, there are only 36. The remaining items are variations on these 36 methods or categories.

Category 12: Consume fewer calories while maintaining your energy expenditure.

On a daily basis, you already burn calories. That's correct! Simply by reading this book, you will burn calories. In fact, when you wake up, breathe, digest food, and pump blood throughout the day, you are burning calories.

Simply put, if your body performs any function, it requires energy. In other words, calories are being burned. This is known as your passive calorie expenditure. If you consume fewer calories than your body requires to function on a daily basis, your body is forced to utilise its stored energy.

In other words, it begins to consume your fat and, eventually, your muscle. This is how it operates. The body must obtain sufficient energy in order to perform its daily functions. When the amount of calories you consume is less than the amount of energy you expend, your body begins to burn fat.

Before you know it, you begin losing weight and improving your appearance.

Category 2: Consume the same number of calories but expend more energy.

You may also choose to invert the situation. When people decide to go to the gym or begin daily physical exercise, they are engaging in this activity. They consume the same amount of food, but engage in more physical activity.

Please recognise that you do not need to overdo it. In terms of physical exertion levels, you do not need to do anything extraordinary. You can expend more energy by walking around the block or a longer distance from the parking lot to your office or school.

The same procedure is repeated. When you consume the same number of calories but expend more energy, your body will seek out alternative energy sources. It initially begins to burn fat and then, eventually, muscle.

The final result is identical. You begin to lose weight.

Category #36: Use both ends of the weight loss candle.

This is common sense. Since you can lose weight simply by consuming fewer calories and expending the same amount of energy, or by consuming the same number of calories and expending more energy, why not do both? This is the third alternative.

Again, this is obvious.

This is typically how weight loss works.

In the grand scheme of things, this is how weight loss typically occurs. It's all about caloric intake and expenditure. This may appear to be a simple task, but the standard American diet makes it difficult for people to accomplish.

Please note that, as a result of modern food technology and transport systems, the typical American diet did not remain confined to the United States. If you are a member of the global middle class, you have probably adopted the standard American diet, which is making you fatter and fatter.just get

Chapter 5: The Impact Of Physical Activity On Body Inflammation

Exercise is one of the most significant factors that can affect inflammation in the body, as previously stated. Depending on how it is performed, exercise can have a positive or negative effect on inflammation. The body mounts an immune response in response to physical stress, just as it would in response to any other potentially harmful stimulus.

The levels of epinephrine, norepinephrine, and cortisol in your blood increase when you begin some form of acute exercise. The hormone epinephrine increases your heart rate and, consequently, the blood flow to your muscles. Norepinephrine is the hormone responsible for increasing blood pressure, while cortisol, also known as the "stress hormone," raises blood sugar levels. As a result of all these hormones acting on your muscles, they will soon feel sore, tired, or numb, as they have become inflamed. Thus, exercise will temporarily increase inflammation.

However, if you allow your body to rest completely after exercise, other hormones such as testosterone and growth hormone will take over, while epinephrine, norepinephrine, and cortisol levels decrease. A large amount of testosterone and growth hormone will be secreted, and they will aid in the repair of damaged muscles and other tissues, facilitating a speedy recovery. Muscle cells will develop that are capable of withstanding significantly more force than they could initially. The more you exercise and rest adequately between bouts of exercise, the more muscle mass is built and the stronger these muscles become. As a result, performing the action would be less of a strain on the body, and less of the hormones described in the preceding paragraph would be secreted. Therefore, exercise with sufficient rest periods in between reduces inflammation over the long term.

But what happens when you consistently place your body under stress by exercising without allowing it sufficient time to recover? Well, rather than reducing inflammation over time, this type of exercise would actually increase it! Your body would be in a constant state of inflammation, and your stress hormones would soar. Instead of healing and becoming even more powerful, your muscles would become even more sore and weaker. Therefore, the next time you engage in some form of exercise, your body will be subjected to greater stress, resulting in a greater release of stress hormones. Overall, you would be degrading your body's tissues, and your body was not designed to withstand a prolonged state of heightened inflammation; therefore, no matter how hard you try, you would not lose the weight that you so desperately really want to lose.

Therefore, it is imperative that you monitor the quantity and intensity of your exercise. In the sections that follow, I will teach you precisely how to do this in a foolproof manner, so that you can easily maximise your exercise programme, finally lose weight, and just keep it off as well.simply put simply put really want just get just keep

Chapter 6: Imagine New Dreams

Welcome to the dream field. The place where you will be reborn as the person you hope to become, reborn in the flames of your imagination. Here, you are expected to express your emotions freely. In this field of manifestation, you will visualise the individual you wish to become in the future. You have channelled your energy and used it to erase the pain of your past and to diminish the impact of negative words. The subsequent step is to create. This field of dreams in front of you is intended to inspire you and inject a great deal of positive energy into your creative process.

Therefore, this next step will be taken in three phases. The initial phase will consist of absorbing the energy that animates the field of dreams. Then, you will visualise the person you aspire to be and the life you would lead. In the third phase, you will invoke the existence of that life. This exercise, as well as every other exercise you've attempted, is crucial to your progress. It requires mental steadiness and a strong sense of purpose. Just keep your mind uncluttered and undistracted. Concentrate on what you will do next. Observe the tone of my voice. Just keep your breathing calm but robust. Maintain your current rhythm. Maintain the same pace. Inhale deeply followed by a slow exhale.

Phase 12 requires you to absorb the energy present in the dream field. The energy is composed entirely of light. It enables you to be creative. It is brimming with inspiration, hope, and fierce resolve. It does not acknowledge or care about the nature of your current situation. Instead, it will bend the situation to your will. It blurs the distinction between your desires and the tragedies you have endured in life. Here, it makes no difference who you are or were. Fate has no influence over what a person can become. You have control over the outcomes of your future experiences. You may have been inhibited by shyness, fear of failure, and anxiety, which have rendered you socially inept. In the realm of dreams, none of this is relevant.

Therefore, realise that right now, your will and courage will deliver the dreams you wish to manifest. Leave regrets and fears behind. Leave worry and anxiety behind. Determine to be strong. Will yourself to be courageous. Will your inner being become courageous? Determine within yourself to bind your self-confidence and faith to the surrounding light. Thus, whenever you feel helpless, exploited, or manipulated, you gain the ability to circumvent such situations. The field of dreams provides you with charisma, intelligence, and bravery. Open your heart to the waves of energy that are pulsating all around you, keeping in mind all the information I have shared.

Permit this powerful energy to pass through you. It is present in the air you breathe. The wind is what touches your skin. And as you continue to inhale and exhale, you acquire all the energy necessary to dream new dreams. Inhale deeply. Embrace the creative powers that are currently flowing through you.

Exhale gradually. Release your anger and any energy that will oppose the thoughts you are about to will into existence. Inhale deeply. Let your shoulders relax. Stay in the present moment. Focus on the sound of your voice and the rhythm of your breathing to anchor yourself to the field of dreams. Continue in this manner. You are in the proper location at the proper time. Everything will work out to your advantage.

In phase two, we will discuss the individual you wish to become and the legacy you wish to leave behind. When constructing your new self, you must separate wishful thinking based on unsubstantial factors. You may decide that you really want to become a billionaire, for instance. This will only be wishful thinking if it is not based on character traits that will manifest the desired outcome. In essence, if you wish to be confident, you should consider the personal actions that will help you manifest confidence. The initial step is to declare your intention. You intend to genuinely enjoy people's company and to be able to express your thoughts freely, clearly, and accurately.

With your intentions clearly articulated, you have established the correct blueprint for creating the person you really want to become and how that person will live in the future. Take a full breath in. Allow it to fill your lungs and enter your abdomen. Just keep it in the centre of your stomach. Slowly exhale and allow your body to unwind as the air leaves your lungs. Repeat this procedure while maintaining a steady rhythm. Imagine a tall mirror standing in front of you at this moment. In and around the mirror, the light emitted by the energy you have absorbed is visible. Look into the surface of the mirror. You would see a reflection of yourself... not as you are currently, but as the person you aspire to be. Attend to the particulars.

Consider how you stand. The vigour of your posture should exude assurance. Pay close attention to your appearance. How you dress is both a reflection of your personal style and a declaration of how you really want others to perceive you. Add to the image what you desire and remove what you do not like. Just keep this image in your mind because you will need it for the next exercise. Modify this reflection of yourself without external influence as much as possible. Building confidence does not require a car, a home, or a partner. They may boost your confidence, but it is a false sense of security. Concentrate on yourself. Adjust your reflection's appearance until you are satisfied.

Now that you have a clear vision of the person you wish to project to the world, you must use the energy you have absorbed from the field of dreams to purify and manifest that image. Remove any doubts you have about your strength from your mind. Establish yourself in the image of your new self. Inscribe the memory of your new dreams in your mind's eye. Consider the new experiences you will have in social situations. Your days of social discomfort and embarrassment are over. You are an excellent candidate for any social environment. Regardless of the social event in which you currently find yourself, you will be a welcome participant going forward. Whether at a public event or in a private conversation, your future encounters will be positive.really want really want Just keep Just keep really want really want really want really want really want really want really want Just keep really want

Chapter 7: How To Lose Weight On The Bulletproof Diet And Crucial Supplement Information

When it comes to weight loss with the Bulletproof Diet, a large number of people have achieved significant results. Many are surprised by their own results. Why is this individual losing so much weight? This is because the Bullet Proof Diet is a lifestyle. Combined with exercise and an active lifestyle, the Bullet Proof Diet can help you achieve a healthy weight and promote muscle growth.

The Bullet Proof Diet is not a miraculous programme. It emphasises only what your body actually requires and avoids most of what it does not.

The Bullet Proof Diet does not prohibit you from consuming your favourite foods, only that you must consume them in moderation. Additionally, it emphasises that you should not deny yourself something you enjoy; rather, you should monitor how much of it you consume. How about that as a diet? You can still enjoy your favourite foods!

The best aspect of the Bullet Proof Diet is that it does not require daily diet pills. The primary focus of your diet is what you eat and how you prepare it, or don't prepare it. We are all aware that raw fruits and vegetables are the healthiest for us, and the Bullet Proof Diet emphasises this fact, which we already know. There are no surprises, and there is no extra time spent studying things that are uncertain. Best of all, guessing games are eliminated.

Why spend hours searching for the ideal diet when all you need to do is consume natural foods in their natural state?

Certain foods, such as meat, must be cooked, but knowing to what extent you must easy cook the meat will also help you improve your health, lose weight, and prevent future disease and illness.

What You Can Expect While Following The Bulletproof Diet

We are all aware of how challenging it is for our bodies to adapt to dietary changes. Not only from a mental standpoint, but also in terms of your body adjusting to foods that are easier to digest.

While your body adapts to necessary dietary changes, such as the Bulletproof diet, you may experience normal abdominal discomfort. This means that you may need to make a few additional trips to the bathroom from time to time. Why is this occurring? Your body is attempting to adapt to a much healthier lifestyle and is flushing out any excess fats you have managed to store.

While it may take some time for your body to adjust to these changes, it will ultimately be beneficial. By adhering to this diet, you make the digestive tract's job much easier and help it conserve energy from over-digesting the harsh foods you once consumed.easy cook easy cook easy cook easy cook

What to Avoid

A healthy, well-balanced diet will provide the immune system with everything it needs to function properly. By substituting unhealthy, processed foods with fresh, nutrient-dense foods, the body will be able to heal and become resistant to disease and infection.

Sugar

Consuming excessive sugar causes stress on the body due to its rapid absorption into the bloodstream and production of insulin. In addition to a variety of health issues, such as type 2 diabetes and brain fog, studies have shown that sugar may displace superior nutrients. This is due to the fact that sugar causes intestinal irritation, which hinders the body's ability to absorb nutrients such as Vitamin C, Vitamin D, Magnesium, and Calcium – all of which are essential for maintaining good health.

Although fruit contains sugar, it also contains fibre, which helps to balance out the sugar. Fruit is also an important source of numerous vitamins that strengthen the immune system and just keep the body healthy.

Conversely, refined sugars found in sweets, chocolate, baked goods, and convenience foods should be avoided because they are addictive and cause the body to desire more. This is due to the rapid absorption into the blood, which causes an almost instantaneous high, followed by a rapid insulin response-induced low. In addition, these foods contain very few essential nutrients and are typically high in calories, which is why they are referred to as "empty calories."

Many individuals assert that they are unable to give up sugar because they have a "sweet tooth" or must eat dessert after a meal. There are many healthier alternatives to refined sugar if this describes you. Numerous sweeteners are composed of artificial ingredients, and while they may be safe, it has been discovered that many of these sweeteners stimulate appetite, which can ultimately lead to overeating and weight gain. Natural sugar substitutes, such as stevia, agave nectar, molasses, and maple syrup, are the best alternatives to sugar.

Sugar addiction is extremely difficult to break and extremely damaging to the body. A weakened immune system can lead to obesity, type 2 diabetes, and other complications. If you have a craving for something sweet, choose a piece of fruit or a healthy smoothie. Your body will thank you.

Caffeine:

Similar to sugar, caffeine is an addictive stimulant with a high potential for abuse. Caffeine, which is found in coffee, tea, energy drinks, and chocolate, temporarily stimulates the central nervous system and induces a feeling of euphoria, but this feeling quickly fades, leaving you feeling exhausted and depressed.

Similar to heroin and cocaine, caffeine increases dopamine levels through a similar mechanism. It injects adrenaline into the bloodstream, giving you a quick burst of energy; however, once this subsides, it often results in a desire for more coffee. This caffeine dependence places stress on the body's organs, which can lead to cardiovascular issues, high blood pressure, and other physical and mental health issues. High caffeine consumption is also directly associated with elevated stress levels, which, as mentioned previously, have a suppressive effect on the immune system.

In addition, caffeine has a diuretic effect, which causes an increase in fluid loss. This can result in dehydration and a loss of water-soluble vitamins, such as vitamin C and B vitamins. Caffeine can also interfere with vitamin D absorption and reduce iron and calcium absorption. Thus, caffeine dependency can contribute to anaemia, osteoporosis, and other nutrient deficiencies. In the following section, vitamins and minerals' immune-supporting properties will be discussed in greater depth.

It is a difficult habit to break if you currently consume a great deal of caffeine. You may experience headaches and fatigue, but rest assured that these symptoms will subside after a few days and that the supplement is doing your body good. Consider some healthier alternatives if you find it difficult to forego your morning cup of coffee. Try green or herbal tea, as it contains little or no caffeine and has some health benefits. If you are unable to give up caffeine, drink it at least two hours before or after a meal to prevent it from interfering with the absorption of nutrients.just get easy cut

Saturated Fats:

It is common knowledge that saturated fats are unhealthy and must be avoided whenever possible. However, in the Western world, many foods contain concealed saturated fats, making it difficult to avoid them. This is typically a problem, particularly with highly processed foods like fast food, convenience foods, and frozen meals.

According to a recent study, saturated fats begin to harm the immune system prior to weight gain. This is due to the fact that excessive consumption of saturated fats is a form of malnutrition, which causes the immune system to attack healthy parts of the body, in some cases resulting in autoimmune diseases such as type 12 diabetes, rheumatoid arthritis, and inflammatory bowel disease. The compromised immune system leaves the body susceptible to infections, diseases, and viruses.

The best way to reduce consumption of saturated fat is to consume a plant-based diet rich in whole foods. This is one of the world's healthiest diets, as it excludes processed and junk foods while emphasising whole grains, fruits, vegetables, legumes, and small amounts of healthy fats from nuts and seeds. The benefits of a whole-food, plant-based diet should not be overlooked, despite the fact that many people may view it as extreme. Due to the nutritional profile of the foods involved, it has been linked to a longer life expectancy, a reduced risk of a wide variety of diseases, a lower body mass index, and overall better health.

Smoothie With Cold Brew Colada And Bulletproof Coffee

Ingredients

4 ounces of regular water, or coconut

3 teaspoon of hemp seeds

2 tablespoon of Stevia, or raw honey

2 cup of organic pineapple chunks

12 ounces of light coconut milk, or almond

4 ounces of brewed Bulletproof Coffee, chilled

Directions

Blend the ingredients in a blender until the mixture is completely smooth.

Smoked Salmon And Avocado Are Delectable.

just get Ingredient List:

- 1-5 Pound of Salmon, Smoked Variety and Wild Sockeye Variety
- Dash of Sea Salt, For Taste
- 2 Avocado, Fresh and Peeled

Instructions:

1. Begin by slicing your avocado and salmon into thin strips.
2. Then, wrap slices of avocado around a piece of salmon.
3. Continue until all of the salmon is wrapped.

Season With A Pinch Of Sea Salt And Serve Immediately. Creamy Vegetables

Servings: 2

4 Tbsp. Coconut oil

1 Tbsp. Apple Cider Vinegar

Fresh Herbs Salt to Taste

2 Bunch Asparagus

2 Bunch Broccoli

4 Tbsp. Butter

1. The vegetables should be steamed until tender.
2. While the vegetables are still hot, remove a third of them and puree them in a blender.
3. Together with the remaining ingredients.

To serve, drizzle the dressing over the remaining vegetables.

Grass-Fed Lamb Prepared Moroccan-Style With Sweet And Sour Sprouts.

Ingredients

4tablespoons Moroccan 7 spice.

4cups, Brussel sprouts, halved

Juice of 2 lemon

4table spoon honey

Salt and pepper to taste

3 pounds grass fed lamb shoulder, boned

2 onion, diced

4 clove garlic, minced

Thumb sized piece of ginger, minced

Direction:

1. Add the lamb, onion, ginger, garlic and 7 spice to the slow cooker and easy cook on low heat for 6-6 ½ hours.

2. Once the lamb is cooked, pull apart with a fork and set aside.

3. Lightly boil the Brussels sprouts in water with and drain.

4. Toss with the honey, fresh lemon juice and salt and pepper.

5. Serve alongside the lamb. Drizzle the honey and fresh lemon juices around the plate.

Smoothie With Avocado And Raspberry

Ingredients:

2 cup coconut milk

2 tablespoon MCT oil

8 ice cubes

2 small avocado, peeled and pitted

2 cup fresh raspberries

2 teaspoon lime juice

1 teaspoon lime zest

Directions:

1. Blend all the ingredients until smooth in a blender.

The smoothie should be poured into glasses and served as soon as possible.

Stuffing easy made with Sweet Potatoes

Ingredients

10 diced sweet potatoes

6 Tbsp. mixed herbs – Mix equal parts – dried or diced fresh

2 Tbsp. cayenne pepper

6 Tbsp. ghee

Chives

Rosemary

Oregano

Parsley

Sage

4 Tbsp. coconut flour

Salt

Directions

1. Heat oven to 450.
2. Simply put diced sweet potatoes in pot and fill with water.
3. Cover and boil. Boil for about 5-10 minutes or until just tender.
4. Place sweet potatoes in bowl of ice water, cool down slightly and drain very well.
5. Simple make sure you just cool off the sweet potatoes here or they will not be crispy later.
6. Place sweet potatoes evenly over a parchment paper lined baking sheet.
7. really do not overcrowd the potatoes.
8. You really want to just get them crispy.

9. Melt ghee in saucepan and drizzle it over the sweet potatoes.

10. Mix the herbs with cayenne pepper.

11. Sprinkle over the sweet potatoes, and toss to coat them.

12. Add coconut flour and toss again.

13. Bake for 35 to 40 minutes or until potatoes just get crispy and brown.

Baked Avocado N' Egg

Ingredients:

Pinch of salt

Pinch of pepper

4 fresh eggs

2 avocado

Direction:

1. Cut Simple halve the avocado along its length and remove the pit.
2. Crack the fresh eggs and place one in the hole of each avocado.
3. They are seasoned with salt and pepper and placed on a baking sheet.
4. Place the baking sheet in the oven and bake at a temperature of 450 °F for approximately 25 to 30 minutes.

Serve without delay.simply put

Guacamole Impenetrable

Ingredients

5-10 tablespoons Upgraded XCT Oil or Brain Octane

2 tablespoons dried organic oregano

8 large ripe Hass avocados, peeled

4 or more teaspoons Himalayan salt

5-10 teaspoons apple cider vinegar

Directions

1. Place all the ingredients in your blender and blend until very creamy. If you want, add some chopped cilantro or any other herbs you really want and stir.

2. This guacamole recipe that is extremely tasty will just keep you satiated.
3. Try it in sushi, grass-fed meats or salads.
4. Save some for tomorrow's lunch.

Gluten-free Crepes

Ingredients:

- ½ teaspoon baking soda
- ½ teaspoon sea salt
- 2 tablespoon coconut oil or grass fed unsalted butter melted + extra for greasing
- 3 cups almond meal
- 12 tablespoons almond milk, unsweetened
- 4 small pastured fresh eggs
- 1 tablespoon ground flaxseed

Direction:

1. Whisk together fresh eggs and almond milk in a large bowl.
2. Add oil or butter and whisk well.

3. Mix together all the dry ingredients in a bowl and add to the fresh egg mixture little by little, whisking each time.

4. Add more milk if you find the batter too thick.

5. Add a tablespoon at a time and whisk.

6. Place a nonstick skillet over medium heat.

7. Grease the pan.

8. Pour about ½ cup batter on the pan.

9. Slightly swirl the pan so that the batter spreads.

10. Easy cook until the underside is golden brown.

11. Flip sides and easy cook the other side too.

12. Repeat steps 10-15 with the remaining batter. It makes about 10-15 pancakes
13. Serve with yogurt and fresh fruits.

Coffee Made With Coconut Butter
Ingredients:

- 4 tbsp coconut butter
- 2 tbsp sugar-free maple syrup
- 2 cup freshly brewed coffee

Instructions:
Blend all the ingredients until smooth and pour into a serving glass.
2. Enjoy!

Fat bombs

10 g grated coconut

10 g coconut oil, for chocolate

100 g bitter chocolate (dark)

100 g unsalted butter

500 g cream cheese

1 lemon, juice and zest

Preparation:

1. Prepare 2 2 small silicone molds or line a 20x20 cm (8x8 ") square mold with parchment paper, to facilitate demoulding.
2. Melt the butter and coconut oil in the microwave, at intervals of 25 to 30 sec.
3. Add the cream cheese and mix well. Add the lemon juice and zest and the grated coconut, mix.
4. Spread the mixture in the mold.
5. Melt the chocolate and coconut oil in the microwave at 50-90 second intervals.
6. Spread over the cream cheese mixture.
7. Refrigerate until solid, about 2 hr.

8. Unmold onto a work surface and remove the paper.
9. Easy cut into squares to obtain 1-5 pieces.

Buttery Broccoli

Ingredients:

1/2   cup unsalted butter, melted

2   large   broccoli

Method:

1. Rinse the broccoli, pat it dry and trim it. Separate the florets and set aside.

2. Simply put water and a pinch of salt in a pan. Bring the water to a boil and add the broccoli florets to the pan.

3. Easy cook the broccoli until color becomes bright green.

4. Transfer the broccoli on paper towels to absorb excess liquid.

5. Simply put the broccoli florets in a bowl, pour the melted butter over them and then toss to coat.

Vanilla Cream Bulletproof

Ingredients:

- 2 tsp vanilla extract
- 2 tbsp without sugar maple syrup
- 2 tbsp unsalted butter

- 3 cups newly fermented coffee
- 2 tbsp MCT oil
- 4 tbsp weighty cream

Instructions:

1. Process every one of the fixings in a blender until smooth.
2. Fill a spotless glass and enjoy.

'Whatever' Exclaimed Tor Dnner

Ingredients:

- 2 'green zone' meat
- 1-5 'green zone' vegetables, chopped
- spinach or kale
- your choice herbs/spices

Directions:

1. Simply put some coconut oil in a pan on medium heat.
2. Lightly brown the meat and then
3. add the vfresh egg ies and your leafy greens. Sprinkle in your spices and herbs. Stir,
4. cover, and let it cook until veggies are tender, usually 20 to 25 minutes.

Cauliflower Curry

Ingredients:

½ cup water
2 teaspoon curry powder

2 head cauliflower
2 cup coconut milk

2 tablespoons cashews chopped:

1. Rinse cauliflower with water and pat dry. Trim and separate the cauliflower florets.
2. Put Simply combine the florets, cashews, coconut milk, and water in a saucepan and cook on low heat for 20 minutes.

Remove the pan from the heat and mash the cauliflower with a fork. Before serving, season it with curry and a pinch of salt.

Sausage-Burger Balls

Ingredients:

1 lb. spicy sausage or chorizo

1 lb. ground beef

2 fresh egg

oregano or basil (to taste)

Directions:

1. Preheat oven to 350 degrees F. In a large bowl, mix all the ingredients.
2. Form the mixture into bite-sized mini-meatballs.
3. Easy cook in a flat baking dish with sides until desired doneness is reached, about 25 to 30 minutes.

Eggs Scrambled With Spinach

Ingredients:

4 cloves garlic, minced
4 red onions, diced
1 teaspoon dried oregano Pinch of salt, pinch of pepper

12 fresh eggs
1000 grams ground beef
4 cups spinach
4 tablespoons coconut oil

Direction:

1. Trim spinach, chop coarsely and then set aside.

2. In a large skillet, heat coconut oil and saute onion and garlic until golden.

3. Add oregano to the skillet and mix ingredients well.

4. Season the mixture with salt and pepper.

5. Add the ground beef to the skillet and continue to easy cook for about 10 minutes.

6. Add spinach to the skillet and easy cook for another 1-5 minutes or until wilted.

7. Add beaten fresh eggs to the mixture, stir, and continue to easy

cook for about 1-5 minutes or until set.

Watercress Shake

Ingredients:

2 ¾ cups of organic full fat yogurt

Pinch of cayenne pepper

2 large bunch watercress

Direction:

1. Simply put all the ingredients into a blender.

2. Start on a low speed and increase to a high speed.

3. Stop blending when all ingredients are fully blended.

Bulletproof Banana Pancakes

Ingredients:

4 raw pastured fresh eggs

Cinnamon, to taste

2 ripe banana

Preparation:

1. Begin by mashing your banana with a fork in a medium-sized bowl.

2. Combine with fresh eggs and whisk until you achieve a smooth consistency.

3. Easy cook on a griddle or in a skillet on the stovetop, easily making sure that each side is golden-brown and thoroughly heated.

www.ingramcontent.com/pod-product-compliance
Lightning Source LLC
LaVergne TN
LVHW011737060526
838200LV00051B/3213